"God provides the wind, but man must raise the sails."

— St. Augustine

Dedicated to the memory of my father, Sam Bayer,
who mastered the art of saving money and taught me
this wisdom as well.

Heaven on on Earth Publishing
Bayer Communications
169 Plochman Lane
Woodstock, NY 12498

Design: Avenue C Productions
Cover Illustration: Margaret Tanzosh

THE PROSPERITY AEROBICS:

Mental Exercises To Increase Money Flow and Success

Cary Bayer

HEAVEN ON EARTH PUBLISHING

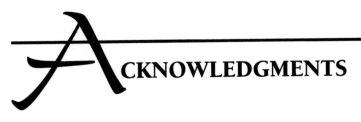

ACKNOWLEDGMENTS

I'd like to thank Fred Lehrman, whose wonderful workshop, "The Psychology of Wealth: Getting Money Right," changed my life. Most of all it made me realize that our thoughts—even the ones that aren't conscious—have a profound effect on our money supply.

Kudos to Phil Laut for his outstanding "Money is My Friend" seminar and book. And thanks for saying it was time to lead a seminar.

Gratitude to Bob Mandel, as well, for his brilliant concept of the personalized Money Mantra, and for a keen sense of humor which has inspired how I lead my own seminars.

Foster Hibbard's boundless enthusiasm has energized my work and given me a taste of what it must have been like studying with Napoleon Hill. Thanks for that gift.

Peter Fein for telling me it was time to write this book.

Jeff Williamson of Avenue C Productions, a long-time pal who's now my desktop publisher.

David Goldbeck for his book publishing tips.

Morry Fraid, an enormously prosperous and generous Aussie who lives life as if it were one endless g'day.

Sharon Nichols for some chapter titles, Kerry Mauldin-Moskowitz for some word processing.

Most of all I'd like to thank Barbara Bayer, my mate, confidante, editor and better half, especially when it comes to spending money. She helps make having money a lot more fun.

"Allow yourself to have desires in order to observe the Tao's manifestations."

— Lao Tzu, *Tao Te Ching*

C ONTENTS

"A feast is made for laughter, and wine maketh merry but money answereth all things."

— Ecclesiastes (10:19)

"You can go to the ocean with a teaspoon or a bucket, the ocean doesn't care."

— Rev. Ike

WARM UP: INTRODUCTION

Aerobics are physical exercises that help oxygen flow better in the body, get the heart functioning optimally and strengthen the various muscle groups that are being worked out.

So what then are "prosperity" aerobics? In short, they are mental, emotional, perceptual and physical activities that strengthen the various mental and emotional muscles, if you will, that help us prosper in this life. Some of these exercises also strengthen our heart—but in a much different way than running in place does. Cardiologists haven't figured out how to measure purity of heart just yet.

Our own state of mind, the quality of our relationships, our ability to conceive success—all of these play a major factor in how much success and prosperity actually dawn in our lives. The Prosperity Aerobics, therefore, is a program of processes—some of which are done daily, others which are done just once—designed to enliven and tone these mental and emotional muscles. The stronger and more toned the muscles, the more success and prosperity we can draw to us.

Gold's Gym helps tone the body and strengthen muscles; the Prosperity Aerobics will transform the mind into a gym in which gold can be mined.

Oh...and there's one other nice feature of these aerobics. There's almost no pain—yet an abundance to gain! Mix up the daily routine of exercises outlined in the book but make sure you do a good 15 minutes at least every day. There is so much negativity that the world is ready to dump on you each day, the least you can do is spend a quarter of an hour a day to offset that. Start erasing negative tapes learned in childhood and make yourself a powerful generator of positivity.

1

"There is a certain Buddhistic calm that comes with having...money in the bank."

— Tom Robbins

CHAPTER 1

SPIRIT LIFT: CREATING A BUSINESS BASED ON FUN

"If you're not doing God's work, find another employer."

—Phil Laut

1. Take 2 minutes and write down your 10 favorite pleasures.

2. Review the list and select the very favorite pleasure that you are willing to receive money for.

3. Take 2 minutes and make a list of 10 ways that you can provide a service for people by performing your very favorite pleasure that you are willing to receive money for. Remember: you have to be willing to be paid for this pleasure-turned-service.

4. Review the list you just wrote and pick out your favorite way of providing a service for people. What you have before you now is your very favorite money-making idea.

5. Take another 2 minutes to make a list of 10 things that you are willing to do to make your favorite money-making idea into a financial success.

6. This is the important question: Are you now willing to see this favorite money-making idea turn into a success? Are you willing to do what it takes to make at least $100? If not, go back to step 1.

7. Start implementing your pleasurable business and enjoy.

Source: Phil Laut, *Money is My Friend*

"Work is love made visible."

— Kahlil Gibran

CHAPTER 2

INNER MUSCLE TONING: AFFIRMATIONS

The English word "affirmation" comes from the Latin word affirmare, which means to make firm or to fix. And the way it's made firm in the mind is through repetition. That's the way we learn anything, the way those who use mantras transform consciousness.

An affirmation is a powerful thought — something you aspire to — which is planted in the fertile soil of consciousness to germinate into reality.

Let's say the affirmation is, "It's holy to prosper," a thought that was recognized as an indisputable truth by people in the days of Abraham, Isaac and Jacob. They understood that prosperity was a blessing from God. But today, millions of people think "spiritual" people and artists should struggle materially. Using such an affirmation could work wonders in transforming their understanding.

The Prosperity Aerobics recommends using affirmations so that they work on three senses: sight, hearing and touch.

HEARING

To hear affirmations, I highly recommend taking many or all of the affirmations in this book and putting them on tape in your own voice. Alternate with first person, second person and third person.

So if the affirmation is: My income now and always exceeds my expenses, I would record it the following way on tape:

My income now and always exceeds my expenses.

*Y*our income, *C*ary, now and always exceeds your expenses.

*C*ary's income now and always exceeds his expenses.

SEEING

It's good to post some of these affirmations in places where you'll see them: in the mirror, on the fridge, at your desk, by your bed, etc.

TOUCHING

Personally, I think the best way to use the affirmations in this book is through writing. And the best way to do that is to divide the page in half. At the left margin, write the affirmation. At the middle of the page write the response that comes up in your mind as you write the affirmation.

So if the affirmation is, "My income now and always exceeds my expenses," and the thought you have while writing it is something like "Fat chance!" or "Give me a break; I'm a month from bankruptcy," write that response.

This process honors the material that rises from the unconscious that is in opposition to the affirmation. Such material is there in abundance—if it weren't you wouldn't need to be working with the affirmation that brought it up in the first place. Writing the response is like releasing the resistance from your being. I recommend writing these affirmations 10 times a day for a week.

EARNING AFFIRMATIONS

I now make an abundance of money doing the things I love.

My job is the pipeline by which I tap the infinite wealth of the U.S. economy for my own personal desires.

I can earn money doing the things I enjoy most.

It's innocent to receive.

I deserve to be wealthy.

God is my unfailing supply. Large sums of money come to me quickly under grace in perfect ways.

SAVING AFFIRMATIONS

The first part of all I earn is mine to keep.

My income increases every day whether I'm working, sleeping or playing.

It's pleasurable and easy to save money.

My income now and always greatly exceeds my expenses.

Spending Affirmations

Since my income always exceeds my expenses, it's a pleasure to spend money within my means.

I always pay my credit card bills in full and on time.

Every dollar I spend comes back to me multiplied.

I pay all my bills promptly.

Investing Affirmations

All my investments are profitable.

Part of all my profits goes into permanent wealth, current expenses, capital and reserves.

I only invest in winners.

> *"The two most beautiful words in the language: 'Check enclosed.'"*
>
> — Dorothy Parker

"Don't try. Do or don't do."

— Yoda, "The Empire Strikes Back"

CHAPTER 3

MIRROR STARE MASTER

Some of the most successful leaders of the 20th Century have had more adventures with the mirror than Alice. Foster Hibbard said that his teacher, Napoleon Hill, claimed that great leaders like Winston Churchill, Teddy Roosevelt and Woodrow Wilson all derived great results from their work in front of the glass.

The process they employed is simple: look into the mirror when you're by yourself and speak energetically and enthusiastically to the reflection that you see. While the words spoken may vary from one person to another, two of the most powerful to use are:

"Get Excited!"

and

"Enthusiasm!"

Don't much mind the responses that go through your head as you implore your reflection to "Get excited," for example. It's natural to feel foolish at first when you start employing this method in your daily regimen, but in time that self-consciousness will give way to a more confident excited consciousness, a magnetic personality.

It's that kind of enthusiasm in your being, that higher vibration, that will attract more clients and customers to you.

Remember: the English word enthusiasm comes from the Greek word "entheos," defined essentially as a god within.

"I rate enthusiasm even above professional skill. Nothing great was ever achieved without enthusiasm."

— Ralph Waldo Emerson

CHAPTER 4

ENVY RELEASE

Jealousy and envy leave the message that, if we had what the person we envy had, we'd be the subject of jealousy and envy in others. Immediately, our unconscious gets the feeling that it isn't safe to have such a thing, and a further message is registered: stay away from having too much. The good news is that envy and jealousy can be transformed through practice.

One powerful technique taught by former Napoleon Hill student Foster Hibbard is to speak four words when jealousy or envy raise their little green heads.

The four words are:

Now That's For Me!

These words, spoken in relation to whatever elicits the envy, provides a very powerful and positive message to our creative unconscious.

Saying "Now that's for me!" leaves the unmistakable feeling that it's safe to have. In fact, it inspires others to want more as well.

"Father Divine: This is my prayer. I care not what I may permanently possess, but give to me the power to acquire at will whatever I may daily need."

— Swami Kriyananda, *Money Magnetism*

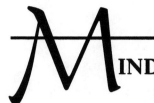IND FIRMING

PART 1

Think this powerful thought 10 times a day:

My mind is a money magnet.

PART 2

Think this powerful thought 10 times a day:

My mind is a money miracle.

PART 3

Think this powerful thought 10 times a day:

My mind is a money machine.

"I built a temple in my inmost mind
  Of pure white marble, its stern
        symmetry
  Became the symbol of tranquility
  How calm it was, and peace, and
        no wind
  Ever disturbed its stillness."

— Paul Mellon

CONSCIOUSNESS RAISE: YOUR MONEY MANTRA

PART 1: THE FAMILY LIE

What you're about to do is first bring to consciousness all the most negative things your Mother and your Father taught you either directly or indirectly about money, work and deserving.

Please bear in mind that as you recall much of this negativity, you may begin to get really angry at your parents for polluting your subconscious with this toxic tape. The purpose of this extremely powerful process is not to get stuck in anger, sadness or self-pity, but to unearth negativity for the purpose of transforming it once and for all into good.

With that said, take out a clean sheet of paper and at the top of it write the following words:

Negative Things My Mother Taught Me About Money and Work

Picture yourself as a small child. Next, visualize your Mother. See if you can remember her telling you about money or about work or jobs or business. Maybe she told you you have to work very long hours to make a living. Perhaps her husband did just that, or was often out of town on business. Perhaps she was in charge of paying the bills and making ends meet. Maybe she didn't do a very good job of it. Maybe she and your Father argued a lot about money, saving it, spending it, investing it.

It's very possible that she never really sat you down and had this kind of chat with you. But something about her behavior spoke volumes. (Remember the old line from Ralph Waldo Emerson: "Who you are speaks so loudly I can't hear what you're saying.") OK, so what did her behavior tell you more covertly?

Did she wear nice clothes or rags? Did she take good care of herself or was she always the last on her list after your Father and her children were provided for? Was she comfortable dealing with money or did she get embarrassed talking about how much she had or didn't have? Was she always speaking negatively about others who had money?

Maybe the messages were something like:

Only men can make money.

Balancing your checkbook and your finances is an utter mystery.

There's never enough money.

Money keeps a family apart.

It takes long hours to make money.

Money is dirty.

You have to do work you hate to take care of a family.

Down the side of the page list some of the negative things you remember learning from your Mother about money and work — whether they were direct or indirect. After jotting down a few (no more than half a dozen) put your pen down.

Then look at your list and put a check mark next to the one that has the most charge for you, the one that somehow most powerfully communicates the most negative thing she taught you about money.

Next, get a clean sheet of paper and duplicate the process, this time recalling what you learned from your Father. Since many of us grew up in families where the father was either the only breadwinner or at least the principal one, you probably learned very different things from him about money and work.

If he hated his job you can be sure he communicated it to you either directly or indirectly. If he had his own business and had a partner or two, or if he owned his own store and had sales help, chances are strong he said something about difficulties trusting them.

So jot down a few of the things Dad taught or communicated indirectly. Then, after writing several of these, put a check mark next to the one that you feel most represents the most negative thoughts about money and work that he communicated to you.

PART 2: DISCOVERING YOUR PERSONAL FAMILY MONEY LIE

In my personal case, the most negative money lesson I learned from my Father was:

"You have to work long hours at jobs you don't like just to make ends meet."

From my Mom I came to understand that:

"Since there's barely enough money to make ends meet, you must spend your money very, very carefully."

Now, if I were to combine each of those sentences into one, we'd get what author and seminar leader Bob Mandel aptly calls the Family Money Lie. In my case it looks like:

"Since you have to work long hours at jobs you don't like just to make ends meet, you must spend your money very, very carefully."

PART 3: YOUR PERSONAL MONEY MANTRA

Your parents generally thought that teaching you the Family Money Lie would best prepare you for the cold, harsh realities of the business world. You can be sure that if they lived through the Depression they always felt—and probably still feel—that an economic crisis could

19

come back again at any time. Lingering recessions can literally terrorize them.

The Personal Money Mantra, which we're about to create now, is the direct opposite of the Family Money Lie. And, truth is, if you somehow were able to tell it to your parents when you were still a small child, they would have thought you crazy, pounded their hearts with a dozen Mea Culpas or sent you to your room without supper. In fact, if you told it to them today their reactions might not be all that different.

To create your Personal Money Mantra simply turn the Family Money Lie completely on its head. Give it a powerful 180 degree spin, until it feels so liberating that you want to go open a bottle of champagne and celebrate.

Let's look at mine and see what you can learn from it to fashion your own. My Family Money Lie, you'll remember, is:

"Since you have to work long hours at jobs you don't like just to make ends meet, you must spend your money very, very carefully."

This is the negative tape that was destined to put me on a frugal lifestyle track, being a workaholic in jobs that underpaid and gave little or no deep personal satisfaction.

Now what about this Personal Money Mantra:

"Since I now make an abundance of money doing things I enjoy, it's fun to spend my money freely."

I remember how liberating it felt when I developed this Money Mantra. This is a powerful affirmation that has made a wonderful difference in my personal life, freeing me to love my work more and start buying $200 shirts I never thought I could "afford" or deserve.

CHAPTER 6

Note in my Personal Money Mantra how the tense used is the present. The word "now" should always be included. Note words like "abundance," "fun," "freely" and "enjoy." These are very liberating for the subconscious. Don't use the future tense, and think big.

I recommend writing the Personal Money Mantra 10 times a day for a month and thinking it 10 times a day until its reality has manifested clearly in your life.

"My boy...always try to run up against money, for if you rub up against money long enough, some of it may rub off on you."

— Damon Runyon

Chapter 7

SUPPORT CIRCLES

Napoleon Hill learned the art of success working, without pay, with one of the most successful people of ours or any century — Andrew Carnegie. Moreover, Carnegie put his young protege in touch with other extraordinary winners of the 20th Century — from Thomas Edison and Henry Ford to Harvey Firestone and Woodrow Wilson.

One of the major lessons Hill learned that you can take advantage of as part of your regular Prosperity Aerobics is the formation and use of a Master Mind.

Hill characterized such a group as a collection of individuals — you might think of anywhere from 5 to 10 people — who are successful in their chosen field of endeavors and who have come together specifically to serve you. Think of it as your personal outside Board of Directors.

The purpose of your Master Mind group is to provide positive support and encouragement of you in your effort to manifest your business plan (see Chapter 1) or making your dream come true. This is a collection of individuals who can keep whatever transpires in these sessions completely confidential, and who can provide practical, prudent and inspirational consultation to the maturation of all plans. You want people who are positive, but grounded and successful. Positive because all new ideas, like newborn babies, are delicate and need nurturing, not discouragement. And successful and grounded so that they can help you make what is ideal real, to turn what is unmanifest into manifestation.

Meeting at least once a month, or hopefully once a week, will exercise your ideas and turn dreams into reality.

Forming a group is easy to do if its purpose is specifically for each member to serve each other member in meetings that are divided up so that all may get their necessary feedback and counsel.

"Hang out with turkeys and you'll be eaten on Thanksgiving. But soar with eagles and you'll be free."

— John Harricharan

CHAPTER 8

VISION STRETCH

One way to let your sense of sight participate in your daily prosperity workout is to create a Treasure Map.

Ingredients:

✓ green or gold construction paper

✓ magazines

✓ travel brochures

✓ photos of yourself

✓ photos of role models who are successes in your chosen field of endeavor

✓ scissors

✓ adhesive tape or glue

Browse through magazines and travel brochures, scissors in hand, cutting out photos and phrases from ads and headlines that inspire you and speak of your prosperity goals.

Include those Ed McMahon letters which say that you have just won $10 million or some such outrageous amount. Cut out those gorgeous pictures of Maui, St. Moritz, or wherever your dream vacation happens to be.

Love those drop dead Beverly Hills pools? Cut one out and tape it on your developing Treasure Map as a visual incentive to manifest it for yourself.

I recommend surrounding yourself with the "Multi Millionaire's Hall of Fame"—photos of people you admire who've already succeeded in the profession of your choice. Writers can surround themselves with best-selling authors they love. Actors are wise to show their favorite star perhaps receiving an Oscar. Painters should be in the company of the artist they love whose work sells for seven, eight and nine figures.

I like to include some upbeat copy in the present tense to illustrate the visuals, such as "Cary is now enjoying his Beverly Hills pool," or "Cary loves to get away to his Parisian pied-a-terre," etc.

The purpose behind Treasure Map creation and daily gazing is to plant images of success into your creative and fertile unconscious. The crop they will eventually harvest will feature many of the images and sentences that you've been gazing upon.

Always be sure to add at the bottom the following line:

This, or something better, now manifests for me in safe and totally harmonious ways for all concerned.

"Begin it now. Until one is committed, there is hesitancy, the chance to draw back, always ineffectiveness. Concerning all acts of initiative (and creation), there is one elementary truth, the ignorance of which kills countless ideas and splendid plans; that the moment one definitely commits oneself, then Providence moves too. All sorts of things occur to help one that would never otherwise have occurred. A whole stream of events issues from the decision, raising in one's favor all manner of unforseen incidents and meetings and material assistance, which no man could have dreamed would have come his way. Whatever you can do or dream you can, begin it. Boldness has genius, power & magic in it. Begin it now!"

— Goethe

*"If the Sun and Moon would doubt
  They'd immediately go out."*

— William Blake

CONTRACTION: HELPLESS DAY

When was the last time you were completely taken care of? I don't mean somebody taking care of your baby while you cook a meal or fix the sink. I mean completely taken care of.

Probably, the last time was when you were sick in bed—and then most likely it was many, many years ago. That's because we're "adulterated," and we don't allow ourselves to get so helpless that someone else has to take care of us. Even when we're sick as a dog, chances are we're still up and about fixing meals for our kids or ourselves, or working in bed.

When we were young, many of us secretly wished we could be sick. Not just so we could stay home from school, but also because our Mom really took care of us.

A Helpless Day is a way for us "adults" to get taken care of without having to get sick. Ideally done with a mate or very close friend (you can even trade Helpless Days), you can relax and let someone else handle all the details for a change.

Want to listen to a particular Mozart CD? Just have your Helpless Day giver take care of it. Want to be read to from *The Mists of Avalon*? Just say the word.

Need a neck or foot massage? No problem. Don't need one, but just want one? Want to have your caregiver literally spoonfeed you the cake in the fridge? Your wish is his/her command.

Depending on your relationship with your caregiver, you could also have a bath or body massage.

The idea isn't to have your own personal slave for a day to do your laundry and scrub your floors, but rather to feel how marvellous it is to let yourself be helpless for a change and be taken care of. This letting go and letting your caregiver provide gives a very powerful message to all those control freaks out there: Namely that you don't have to do it all by yourself. This is a very valuable lesson to learn first hand—especially since none of us (with the possible exception of God) does everything anyway. But those who have a tough time letting go, believe they have to do it all by themselves. Too many of us labor under this ridiculous myth.

Letting another person support you for a day is a powerful demonstration to yourself that you are willing to be supported by others. Becoming successful, after all, is going to require the support of others — their labor, their ideas, their capital.

Being pleasured in such a profound way on your Helpless Day provides an unforgettable firsthand experience: that you, in fact, deserve to have others support you in making your life easier.

"The ideal income is a thousand dollars a day — and expenses."

— Pierre Lorillard

"I am only being a little facetious when I say that in order to be a millionaire all you have to do is learn how to love your parents."

— Phil Laut

FORGIVENESS FLEX

I often think, for all its authority and excellence, the *Wall Street Journal* is derelict in its duty for failing to inform its millions of readers that one of the fastest ways to prosper is to forgive. From my own personal experience, I can assure you that when I've truly forgiven someone against whom I had been holding a great deal of anger, my income grew dramatically.

There was a close relative of mine who stopped talking to me for several years and would return all my letters unopened. Even though I felt deeply wronged by her, I broke the silence and called to apologize for the upset. Within a matter of days I landed the largest account I ever had, and also signed two other clients. It usually took about three months to sign three clients; this time it took about seven days!

FORGIVENESS AEROBICS

PART 1: COMPLETION LETTERS

This process, developed in the Loving Relationships Training (LRT), is a three-part written process, the purpose of which is to "complete" with a particular person for whom you have a great deal of unresolved emotions.

Phase one consists of writing a letter to this person that you never intend to send. In it you tell this person in no uncertain terms, in language barely fit for *cable* television, how you feel about all those horrible things he/she did or didn't do to you. And what a terrible scoundrel or lowlife he/she is. Let it really rip, hold nothing back. In fact, blame the person for just about everything lousy that's ever happened between the two of you. By the time you've finished you'll feel a lot lighter, as if you've let a great weight off your shoulders. Because you have. Then rip up the letter.

Phase two consists of virtually the opposite approach. In it, take a somewhat saintly posture, assuming full responsibility for that evil thing he/she did to you. Get as New Age as you can, thanking the person for presenting this event in your life which you have managed to survive. In fact, you can praise him/her for indirectly showing you just how much self-sufficient survival skills you really have. You're glad to have met this person and experienced this previously huge upset because now you also know first hand how abundant your compassion is. Lay it on thick, be the first Mother Theresa on your block. You're not going to send this letter either.

That brings you to Phase Three, a kind of integration of the first two letters that you didn't send. This note, on the other hand, is intended for the Post Office. By now, you will have released a lot of the venom that you've felt for the person in the first writing, and you will have overdone whatever responsibility you might have for creating the upset you described in letter number two. This will leave you healthy and wise enough to take responsibility for whatever part you might have had in creating the upset, and detached enough to express your pain in a way that the person can hear. It's probably a good idea to have a close friend or therapist look at the letter before you send it to make sure it's ready for the person to read.

Such letters have brought relationships virtually back from the dead. (In fact, it's fine to send this letter to a deceased person, too.) Miracles have come to life out of such communications. And when miracles start happening out of forgiveness, money miracles are usually not far behind.

PART 2: FORGIVENESS DIET

This is a powerful process developed by Sondra Ray, founder of the Loving Relationships Training. Taking a cue from Jesus in the Scriptures, she recommends forgiving a particular person in writing 70 times a day for a period of 7 days.

The line she suggests is,

> I, (your first and last name), now forgive (name of person) completely.

Naturally, start with whomever you hold the most amount of anger towards, but she also recommends doing weekly forgiveness work on your Mother, Father, God, and self. A proponent of Rebirthing, Sondra also recommends forgiveness of your obstetrician, the person who most likely brought you into this world in a less than gentle way.

"Money, which represents the prose of life, and which is hardly spoken of in parlors without an apology, is, in its effects and laws, as beautiful as roses."

— Ralph Waldo Emerson

INCOME RAISE

The following prayer has been used by many people, including myself, with wonderful and surprising results. It's best spoken out loud, once or twice each day, and wonderful in groups dedicated to increasing prosperity.

Enjoy!

The "Unexpected Income!" Prayer

I believe God is the source of all supply, and money is God in action, and should be used for good.

I believe my good is now freely flowing to me so bountifully I cannot use it all, and I have an abundance to spare and to share, today, and always.

I am expecting "Unexpected Income!"

I believe God is now giving this to me and I accept this as Truth and give thanks.

All channels of financial supply are now open to me and I am richly, bountifully and beautifully prospered in every good way.

I believe true Prosperity includes the demonstration of right living conditions, right activity and right kinds of happiness.

This word, which I speak in faith, believing, now activates the law of increased universal good for me and I expect to see rich results now!

I visualize the financial good I expect. I see it coming to me richly and abundantly.

I claim and accept it for myself now.

I am grateful in advance! I bless all the good I now have, and bless the increase.

I bless all others in the "Unexpected Income!" program, and I know we are now all prospering together in every good way, and share the good we receive.

I now freely give my tenth to God's good work. My giving is making me rich!

God gives to me rich, lavish financial blessings now!

This is so now. I am grateful. Thank you, Father!

"You are not a realist unless you believe in miracles."

— Anwar el-Sadat, Nobel Peace Prize-winning
President of Egypt

CHAPTER 12

SUCCESS JOURNAL JOG

Whatever you focus on expands. We hear it all the time. Olympic champions, for example, visualize over and over again their winning performances whether they be on the high bar, the skating rink or in the pool.

Successful people, whether they're in sports or in business, fill their mind's eye with thoughts and images of success.

One way to transform your life from one that fails a lot and succeeds a little into one that succeeds a lot, is to transform your consciousness into a powerful success machine. And an excellent way to do just that is to daily remind yourself of the things that happened that day that were expressions of your Success Consciousness. Perhaps it was a new client you just gained, a wonderful sweepstakes you just won, a lovely present given to you. And it can be small stuff too: the great buys you found at a yard sale that morning, the $1 you found in the street, the cassette tape a friend made for your car. Smaller still for those days where "everything went wrong": the compliment someone paid you for the sweater you wore to the party where your boyfriend found someone else; the nice backhand you hit in a 6-0, 6-0 trouncing you took on the tennis court; your courage to keep going on for another day even though your life is collapsing around you.

This process is ideally done at the end of the day before going to bed, and usually takes no more than two minutes. When you find that it's taking you 10 minutes to do because your day is filled with so much success, either grin and bear it, developing an even stronger success consciousness or rejoice: you're a veritable success machine and you no longer need to keep reminding yourself of the obvious.

"*I've never been poor, only broke. Being poor is a frame of mind. Being broke is a temporary situation.*"

— Mike Todd

THE BANK VAULT: MULTI-ACCOUNTS SAVINGS

While it's historically obvious that one can make far greater money investing in the stock markets than by putting savings in bank accounts, the low rate of savings in this country is frightening, and readers would be wise to master savings through this enlightened approach to using the banking system. As then-President Bush put it succinctly, "Americans need to learn how to save."

All too often, the only bank account that an individual or a family has is a checking account. The problem with this is that the purpose of a checking account is to spend money, not to save it. Electronically linking several specific savings accounts to that checking account will do wonders for your Prosperity Consciousness.

You might wonder why *several* accounts. To which I say, remember the old Christmas club account? That was a specialized savings plan that you contributed to regularly so that by a given time (each Christmas) the account was well stocked to handle your Christmas gift giving.

Imagine a vacation account that works the same way. When summer comes, the money that's needed to travel is now mysteriously there. Except there's nothing mysterious to it — it's just good old-fashioned discipline and making conscious choices that made it happen. You no longer have to wrestle with the guilt of taking a vacation when your kids need new clothes. The clothes account pays for clothes, the vacation account handles holidays. Keeping them separate keeps you sane and guilt-free.

A valuable prosperous exercise to practice monthly is to take at least 10 percent of your net income and deposit it among your various savings accounts. Each person will design a roster of accounts that best fits his needs. I used to have 13 accounts—now only five—for such expenses as home improvement, consumer electronics, annual income (enough money to quit your job for a year and live off the money in that account), house down payment, investing (this money goes only into the stock market), and so on.

My favorite account, although it was the most difficult for me at times because of my upbringing in spending carefully, is the impulse spending account. This account should be emptied in full in cash each month, and you shouldn't come home until you've spent it all. The idea will appeal to the child in you who wants what he wants immediately: the first thing you see that you want that costs less than the money you have, you instantly buy. No questions asked, no comparative shopping, no waiting for sales or the store across town. This is also a great way for people who compulsively overspend and incur debt to get what they want regularly—just in a disciplined fashion and within limits. This is the perfect account for those who can save but not spend.

A god-send for those who like to spend but can't save is the financial independence account. This is an account in which you never remove the principal but spend the interest regularly. The idea is to train yourself to live off the interest. This is exactly how many independently wealthy people live—off dividends, but never off their principal.

"I am a great believer in luck, and I find the harder I work, the more I have of it."

— Stephen Leacock

"I've been rich and I've been poor and rich is better."

— Mae West

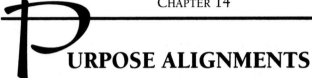

PURPOSE ALIGNMENTS

Those who enjoy writing will like this process. But don't worry, even if you're not much of a writer — perhaps you'd rather walk on hot coals than jot down a few loving thoughts for a birthday or anniversary card — you're going to be glad you did this exercise.

It's time to write the essay of your life, and trust me...you'll love it. Forget about the terror you may have experienced in high school or college at the mere mention of the word essay. Besides, this essay is about your highest aspirations and it's no more than 25 words. So don't be concerned by what you leave out of it, just jot down some things that you do want in it. And don't worry about grammar; nobody's going to grade it.

The essay is called, "My Perfect World." So take about 30 minutes, and no more — because you literally could spend a lifetime writing such a document.

YOUR PERFECT WORLD PROCESS

This is a three-step process which can be done in less than a half hour.

Step 1

On a clean sheet of paper, write down on the top of the page, 10 to 20 things you like about yourself (10 minutes).

Step 2

Then, on a separate sheet, write down 10 to 20 ways you like expressing your favorite characteristics (10 minutes).

Step 3

"The purpose of my life is to use my"

A) Take 3 to 5 of the items you listed in Step 1 by

B) Take 3 to 5 of the items you listed in Step 2
so that

C) Copy your 25-word essay.

What you now have before you is a thumbnail picture of what your perfect world looks like, and what the purpose of your life is. Now go and manifest the purpose of your life.

"Poverty demoralizes…men of sense esteem wealth to be the assimilation of nature to themselves…Power is what they want, not candy-power to execute their design, power to give legs, and feet — form and actuality to their thought; which, to a clear-sighted man, appears the end for which the universe exists…"

— Ralph Waldo Emerson

"Learning to sell is far easier than commuting."

— Phil Laut

CHAPTER 15

SELLING THRUSTS

One technique that I learned from Phil Laut, author of the fabulous book, *Money is My Friend*, that I couldn't recommend more highly, is to get into the habit of selling something all the time.

Phil would say find something you can get inexpensively, perhaps at wholesale prices, that you could sell for $1 or $2. Show it to people at parties, on busses or trains, and take it with you wherever you go. As you get good at selling it, move on to something double the price that you like. And when that is moving nicely find something else for double that price.

In time, people will come to see you as a portable store, a veritable selling machine. While it's true you won't get rich selling $5 items (though don't tell that to Sam Walton), your success at selling small items will be of immeasurable value in your ability to negotiate a nice raise, land a $25,000 client or sign a multi-million dollar contract for that matter.

In fact, Phil told me he gave this very advice to a large real estate brokerage firm that often sold $1-million properties. They laughed, saying how could selling a $2 pen help them in moving $1-million estates? Phil's reply: selling is selling. And the more comfortable you get in handling the fears of rejection on $1 deals, the more you can handle the feelings that come up on $1-million deals. Selling, Phil noted, is about 90% dealing with the feelings that come up. Deal with them daily on a small scale and your success will grow on the bigger stuff.

"The lack of money is the root of all evil."

— George Bernard Shaw

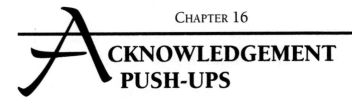

CHAPTER 16

ACKNOWLEDGEMENT PUSH-UPS

A wonderful way of adding to your prosperity consciousness for those who live with another person (mate, parent, child, friend, roommate, etc.) is to have that person praise you nightly for a minute or two. This is a variation of the process of writing in your success diary nightly that was previously described, except that in this case it's verbal and it's done by someone other than yourself.

Simply have that person fill in the blank,

"Something I want to acknowledge about your prosperity and success is ..."

After they say one such acknowledgement, you simply say, "Thank you."

Don't get into a big conversation, and definitely don't deny any of these compliments. Just take it in with a breath and a thank you.

And have your partner in the process repeat another one, "Something I want to acknowledge about your prosperity and success is ..."

It couldn't hurt to return the favor to your partner by praising him/her in the area of his/her life that he/she chooses to stimulate, be it health, sexuality, relationships, etc.

"God desires ease for you and desires not hardship."

— The Koran

ENEROSITY STRETCHES: TITHING

It's as ancient as the hills of Judea, and truly one of the most powerful prospering practices there is. Called tithing in the Old Testament, it has been used by millions of people throughout the world as a way of expressing gratitude to the Highest Power of the universe.

In *The Seven Against Thebes*, the great Greek playwright Aeschylus wrote that a state that is prosperous always honors the gods.

Tithing is the act of giving 10 percent of your income to those organizations or people who do the work of the Highest Power of the Universe. And those who do it have been delighted to enjoy the way increased income results.

Abraham, Isaac, Jacob, Joseph, Moses and most of the ancient Hebrew people portrayed in the Bible were regular tithers. And they were still giving 10 percent or more to the Temple when Jesus was growing up learning Jewish law. The early Patriarchs were extremely wealthy people who understood that the source of their wealth was their God. Honoring this Higher Power that gave them the ability to prosper enabled them to prosper even more. After their prayers were answered the ancients built altars to God. More precisely, they often did "faith offerings" after a prayer was made and "thanks offerings" after a prayer was answered.

The Bible is absolutely clear on this point: "Thou shalt remember Jehovah, thy God, for it is He that giveth thee power to get wealth." (Deuteronomy, 8:18)

Elsewhere, we read, "Bring the full tithes into the storehouse, that there may be food in my house, and thereby put me to the test, says the Lord of hosts, if I will not open the windows of heaven for you and pour down for you an overflowing blessing." (Malachi, 3:10)

CHAPTER 17

Jacob, one of two sons of the great Hebrew Patriarch Isaac, understood that the tithe was a 10% figure. Consider the words that he spoke to his God: "Of all that Thou shalt give me, I will surely give the tenth unto Thee." (Genesis, 28:20)

Since God is the giver of all gifts, not tithing is like stealing, say many prosperity masters. In India, the act of honoring the invisible Source of Life for what one has been given was also widely known. In his commentary on the *Bhagavad-Gita*, the scripture of Yoga, Maharishi Mahesh Yogi wrote quite clearly about this point about stealing: "He who enjoys their (Nature's) gifts without offering to them is merely a thief."

Tithing may feel like a giant risk if you've never done it, but it's a remarkably powerful process. Try it, you'll thrive on it.

"Prosperity is the blessing of the Old Testament."

— Sir Francis Bacon

"Only when a man's life comes to its end in prosperity dare we call him happy."

— Aeschylus

CHAPTER 18

CREDITOR JUMP

We learned in the previous chapter how it pays, from the standpoint of universal laws, to give. In this chapter we will see how we can begin prospering by learning to pay for things quickly.

There are several advantages to paying for things promptly, the least of which is to save enormous amounts of money. More on this in a little while. But first things first. A word to those who let their bills pile up in their in-boxes or, worse, in their drawer somewhere under photographs and those articles from last year's magazines that they meant to read when they had a moment. Or for those who don't even bother to open their bills.

Pay your bills when you get them. Sure, most suppliers of services like rent/mortgage, heating/oil, phone company, cable, etc. give you some time to pay their invoices, ultimately giving you more time to creatively let your money make more money for yourself instead of them. So if you know how to use the float and be creative with your money this way, this point may not apply to you — just make sure to pay the bill before being penalized for late fees. But the majority of people reading this book would be far better served by creating in their consciousness the realization that they never have bills to pay (because they've already paid them) rather than the nagging stressful burden of always having bills to pay (because they never get around to paying them on time). Procrastination also runs the risk of having to pay penalties, especially if the bill is for the mortgage or a credit card. (Those late fees, called service charges, *really* hurt.)

Those who are on a program to pay off large amounts of secured debt (like a mortgage or a car payment, etc.) are wise to pre-pay the principal whenever possible. In other words, pay off more than the amount you are supposed to pay and you will save a small fortune. In his eye-opening book, *The Banker's Secret*, consumer advocate Marc Eisenson says that on a $75,000 loan, taken at 10% interest for 30 years, one would wind up paying $162,000 *in interest alone*. Yipes! That means, a $100,000 house that you managed to scrape together 25% down payment on would cost $237,000 — not the $100,000 you thought you were getting it for.

On the other hand, if you paid just $25 a month extra (one dinner out for a couple) which you applied to the principal for the term of the loan, you would save more than $34,000 — and the house would be yours free and clear 5 years and 3 months sooner. (That's 63 monthly payments you won't have to be bothered with.)

Suppose, for example, either through increased income, better managing or a little more common sense frugality, you could send in an extra $100 per month applied toward pre-payment of the loan, instead of the $25 we cited above. By the time the loan had been retired you'd be $78,000 richer than if you had quietly gone ahead and made each mortgage payment the way your booklet said. And the house would be all yours — and not the bank's — in 17 ½ years — not 30.

Exercise your choice. But if you're opting for Prosperity Aerobics, I think I know which way you'll go. A little bit of knowledge can be extremely liberating.

"...the philosophers have laid the greatness of man in making his wants few, but will a man content himself with a hut and a handful of dried peas? He is born to be rich... Wealth requires — besides the crust of bread and the roof — the freedom of the city, the freedom of the earth, travelling, machinery, the benefits of science, and fine arts, the best culture and the best company. He is the rich man who can avail himself of all men's faculties."

— Ralph Waldo Emerson

"Almost any man knows how to earn money, but not one in a million knows how to spend it."

— Henry David Thoreau

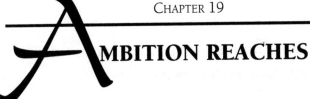

CHAPTER 19

AMBITION REACHES

Exercise your imagination and exorcise your lethargy. As the tv show was so aptly named—"This is your life."

Imagine Death knocked on your door and said, "I'm ready to take you if there's nothing else you want to do in life."

Now that would get your juices flowing, wouldn't it? Well, write these lists as if your life depended on it. Because, you know what? It does!

In the course of the next week make a list of 50 things you want to be in life.

Perhaps you'd like to be a husband (wife), a father (mother), a business owner, an author, a playwright, a handyman, a singer, etc. Then start becoming them.

"Your own resolution to succeed is more important than any other one thing."

— Abraham Lincoln

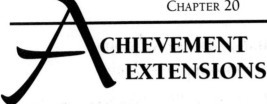CHIEVEMENT EXTENSIONS

"Just do it!"

—Nike

Over the course of the next week, make a list of 50 things you want to do in your life.

Maybe you want to go to Maui, ski the Alps, learn tennis, cook a Chinese meal, speak French, write a book, read a book (this is the video age), deep sea dive, etc. Exercise your desire to do.

Don't ever forget—Death is always knocking on your door when you're not truly living. Looked at another way, the more you do the things you really want to do, the more your life becomes a life really worth living—a life you have no regrets about when Death comes back again and won't take no for an answer.

"The purpose of money is to create the environments within which we can experience the things money can't buy."

— Fredric Lehrman

CHAPTER 21

POSSESSION EXTENSIONS

Now it's time to exercise your desire to have. The more you exercise, the stronger you get.

Perhaps you'd like to own your own home, or second home, or you'd like that Warhol in the gallery you saw on Sunday. Maybe you'd love to drive your own Jaguar, or perhaps it's just to simply buy your own basketball backboard.

The list can clearly go on and on. I'm just asking you to do 50 this week.

"*Life is a checkerboard, and the player opposite you is time. If you hesitate before moving or neglect to move promptly, your men will be wiped off the board by time. You are playing against a partner who will not tolerate indecision.*"

— Napoleon Hill

COOL DOWN: CONCLUSION

Living prosperously is not the end of life but a beginning. Buckminster Fuller used to say that there were enough resources on our planet for every human being to live like a millionaire. That sounds like a pretty prosperous birthright to me.

The Prosperity Aerobics are designed to make a major impact on both your supply of money and your supply of pleasure, well being and overall spirituality. That's because it's a natural series of exercises that taps the almighty power of Nature to support you in fulfilling your life's purposes.

When you find unexpected income from surprising sources, new clients, customers, bonuses, raises and the like, recognize the results of your Prosperity Aerobics workout. When you find yourself in the right place at the right time understand that Nature works invisibly and takes no credit. Just say thank you.

Get used to accepting and saying "Thank you." And that includes when someone wants to give you a free book, a free dinner, a free movie, even a free car. The Universe has zeroes it hasn't even begun to use! When you start tithing and supporting the evolutionary purpose of Nature, get ready for Nature to more than return the favor.

And also get used to enjoying finer things and struggling less. Nature doesn't struggle, and neither will you as you go about fulfilling your unfolding desires. Prosperity author Jerry Gillies told his readers that every time they said they couldn't afford something they wanted they should take out $100 and spend it on themselves. It's an unforgettable way to do fun things and raise your self-worth in the process.

Remember the wonderful thing about adopting the Prosperity Aerobics as a part of your daily workout: it yields no pain and lots of gain.

Enjoy!

"It isn't necessary to be rich and famous to be happy. It's only necessary to be rich."

— Alan Alda

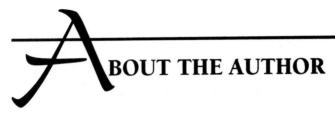# ABOUT THE AUTHOR

Cary Bayer has been leading seminars on personal development in North America and Europe since 1973. His principal topics have included Prosperity, Transcendental Meditation, Rebirthing and Breakthrough Breathing. He currently leads seminars and support groups on the subject of money and prosperity and is available for private consultations, both in person and on the phone.

A business consultant since 1980, he has used his communications skills for David Steinberg and Alan Arkin, Quality Inns, Filippo Berio, Color Tile and Carpet, Wet 'n' Wild and Rolls-Royce of Moscow, among others. He cites as influences an eclectic group that includes Maharishi Mahesh Yogi, Alan Watts, C.G. Jung, Walt Whitman, Herman Hesse, Groucho and Harpo Marx, Superman, Batman and Zorro. His humor has appeared in *Playboy*, the *National Lampoon*, New York's *Daily News* and the *Off the Wall Street Journal* and *Like a Rolling Stone* parodies, and in two humor books that he co-authored: *The Short Report: Good News for Guys 5'7" & Under* and *Fire Island Fried: An Irreverent Guide to an Irreverent Island*. His next book is called "Zen in the Art of Comic Book Heroes."

He currently resides in Woodstock, New York with his wife Barbara and their three cats, Catman, Magic and Ananda.

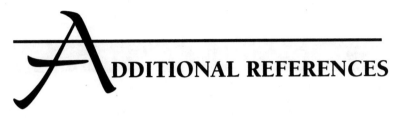

ADDITIONAL REFERENCES

1. Hibbard, Foster, "The Millionaire's Seminar" (Audio Tape Series)

2. Hill, Napoleon, *Think & Grow Rich*

3. Laut, Phil, *Money is My Friend*

4. Lehrman, Fred, "The Psychology of Wealth: Getting Money Right" (Audio Tape Series)

5. Mandel, Bob, *Money Mantras*

6. Mandel, Bob, "Money Mantras" (Audio Tape)

7. Ponder, Catherine, *The Dynamic Laws of Prosperity*

8. Ross, Ruth, *Prospering Woman*

ORDER FORM

Please send me _____ copy(ies) of *The Prosperity Aerobics* **book** by Cary Bayer at $10 each (includes sales tax, postage and handling).

Please send me _____ copy(ies) of *The Prosperity Aerobics* **audio tape** by Cary Bayer at $15 each (includes sales tax, postage and handling).

Please send me _____ copy(ies) of both *The Prosperity Aerobics* **book AND audio tape** by Cary Bayer at the special price of $23 (includes sales tax, postage and handling).

Enclosed please find my check for $_____. Please send the copies to the following address:

NAME _____

ADDRESS _____

_____

Checks should be made payable to Bayer Communications and sent to the following address:

Bayer Communications
169 Plochmann Lane
Woodstock, NY 12498